Daoist Internal Alchemy
And Acupuncture

by

John Orsborn, A.P., D.O.M

Disclaimer:

The information presented in this book does not constitute health or medical advice. It is intended for informational purposes only and is not intended to diagnose, treat, cure, or prevent any condition or disease.

Acknowledgement:

I would like to thank Kenn O'Connor and Rebecca Acosta for their valuable input on the original manuscript.

And a special thank you to my wife, Denise, for always being there. You are my rock, and I love you.

Table of Contents

Introduction

I became interested in Asian culture and the martial arts when I was ten. At that time karate and tae kwan do was what was predominantly taught. These arts are considered external or "hard" martial arts (wài jiā 外家) which rely on physical strength and force against force, similar to boxing. However, I was on the small side and not very athletic. Later, in my teens, I discovered the internal or "soft" martial arts (nèi jiā 內家), like tàijíquán 太極拳 and xíng xì quán 太極拳 which rely more on the practitioner's use of internal energy and meeting opposition without resistance. The concept of "internal energy" fascinated me.

I also became interested in Asian philosophy at this time. I began reading and studying Buddhism, resulting in majoring in philosophy in college. However, the deeper my study of Buddhism went, the more it seemed to me to be mired in human conceptualism, that is, biased by our innate human ability to only understand the world through our limited, human senses, much like most Western philosophy.

A professor then introduced me to Chan (Zen) Buddhism and taught me zazen (Zen meditation). I practiced this meditation and read whatever I could get my hands on; D.T. Suzuki's collected essays, the Mumonkan and the Hekiganroku (the two classical collections of Zen koans or mental riddles), and other books. My journey progressed, my understanding deepened. But yet again, I came to a point where even Chan Buddhism seemed to me to be mired in the human intellectual mind.

One day, in a class on Asian religions (the only way Asian philosophy was taught at that college at that time), the professor said, "Raise your hand if you are the same person right now that you were when you got up this morning." Everyone in the class raised their hand except me. I was thinking of the line from *Alice's Adventures in Wonderland* where Alice states, "… *I know who I was when I got up this morning, but I think I must have been changed several times since then.*" [1] He simply looked at me and smiled, and then we began discussing Daoism.

When I read the opening lines of Gia-fu Feng's translation of the Tao Te Ching (the first of many translations studied over the years), where it says, "The Tao that came be told is not the eternal Tao. The name that can be named is not the eternal name," [2] I was blown away. Here was a philosophical treatise that began by cautioning the reader about the limits of human intellectualism. It began with an admonition stating that what we humans can speak of is only a product of the human mind and not ultimate reality. I have been studying Daoism ever since.

Chinese civilization has been greatly influenced by Daoism. No one can hope to understand Chinese philosophy, religion, government, art, medicine, even cooking, without an appreciation of this profound philosophy. It not only includes doctrines on how to govern and handle daily affairs, but also on cultivating and preserving life. While I have read and studied many of the Daoist alchemical classics, attempting to understand the metaphorical and allegorical terminology, the writings of Zhang Boduan of the Quánzhēn 全真 (Complete Reality) school are what I read most. It wasn't until I began studying Chinese medicine that I began to better understand the language of Daoist internal alchemy.

Chinese medicine is rooted in this tradition. Both are based on the observation of nature and human's place within it. The metaphorical language of the medicine helped me to understand how this philosophy not only influenced the development of the medicine, but how treatments can be based on the concepts of Daoism, especially that of nèidān or internal alchemy. Knowledge of Daoist philosophy is, in my opinion, not only essential to effective treatments, but also to preserving the basis and cultural heritage of this amazing medicine.

The study of Daoism, tàijíquán and qìgōng 气功 for over forty years has been the result of my boyhood interest in internal energy. Being an acupuncture physician for the last fifteen years has furthered my understanding of qi, the vital life force. Attempting to deepen my understanding of Daoist internal alchemy and how classical acupuncture is based on it is now my focus both personally and professionally.

While the principles of Classical Chinese Medicine (CCM) are rooted in Daoist philosophy, especially the Daoist tradition of internal alchemy or neidan 内丹, I have found little contemporary writing on the synthesis of these two traditions. Chinese medicine as it's taught today is referred to as Traditional Chinese Medicine or TCM, which is different from CCM in several ways. Classical Chinese Medicine is based on the philosophical foundation of Chinese culture, which goes back thousands of years. TCM was developed after the fall of the Republic of China in 1949 and, in the U.S. as well as China, is currently taught in accordance to the educational model used in Western biomedical schools. TCM does not focus on the classical writings of Daoist philosophy, or Classical Chinese medicine for that matter, relying more on modern textbooks, most of which are written by individuals who have little to no background in the underlying philosophy upon which this medicine is based.

Chinese medicine is an holistic approach to wellness. The individual is seen as an integral part of nature and all aspects of a person's life are taken into consideration as regards their health. The emphasis is on being and staying healthy, which is more beneficial to the individual and society than waiting until they are sick to find a remedy. One of the metaphorical expressions of this is that it's better to drill a well before one needs water than to wait until one is thirsty.

The goal of this little book is to share my knowledge with anyone who wants to learn about Daoist philosophy, Daoist self-cultivation, and how it is the basis for Classical Chinese medicine. With this knowledge, I hope practitioners who read it will also gain a deeper knowledge of how to further enhance their treatment principles and develop effective treatments. To quote David Hartmann, author of "The Principles and Practical Application of Acupuncture Point Combinations," anyone can be a cook and follow a recipe. A chef creates their own recipes based on their knowledge. Which would you rather be, a cook, or a chef?

Some of the basic concepts in Daoist thought and Chinese history which have influenced acupuncture and Chinese medicine are yang/yin theory, the Wǔ Xíng, the Hé Tú, the Luò Shū, the Nine Palaces, and the Bā Guà. We begin with a discussion of these Daoist philosophical concepts.

Part One – Daoist Philosophy

a. History and Yang/Yin Theory

Daoism is the indigenous, fundamental principle at the center of Chinese philosophical and spiritual thought. It is based on the concept of the Dao 道, which is not easily translated into English. Dao means a way, a path, or a method. I prefer to call it a process. The Dao is the process of nature, the way all things proceed, the way things change. It is the change of night and day, the change of the seasons. It is how life comes to be, flourishes, declines, and ends. Everything in the universe follows the process of the Dao. Ultimately this process cannot be fully known by the human mind, as human conception and cognition are limited in scope. In other words, we humans perceive things in a specifically human way limited by our human senses of perception. However, we can observe patterns in nature and in the human psyche that reflect or mirror the process of the Dao.

The *Dao De Jing* ("The Classic on the Virtue of the Way"), the seminal text of Daoism, is a relatively short book attributed to Lao Zi (Venerable Person), whose real name was Li Er.[3] He was an historian in charge of the Library of Records in Loyang, the capital of the Eastern Zhou dynasty during middle of the Spring and Autumn Period (c. 770 – 476 BCE). It was a time of warfare and governmental corruption. As legend has it, he became disgusted with the affairs of state, so he quit his job and rode off to the west on an ox. According to legend, at a gate in the Zhong Nan mountains, he was detained by the guard who recognized him, and was not allowed passage until he told the guard what he knew about the Dao. This knowledge became the afore mentioned book. He is considered the father of Daoist thought, although these teachings probably predate recorded history.

The basic concept of Daoism is to live in harmony and balance with nature. Humans are a part of nature yet, now days especially, we tend to live apart from nature. To live in harmony and balance with nature, we need to understand the fundamental aspect of life; that change is inevitable and we need to be able to adapt to change. Change is the only constant in life. The only thing that never changes in life is that everything in life changes. The only thing that stays the same is that nothing stays the same. The basic concept of change in Daoism is represented by the concept of yang and yin, a means by which to understand the apparent dichotomy of nature. Yang originally was said to represent the sunny side of a hill and yin the shady side. Thus, yang became associated in part with light, white, heat, activity, heaven, and male, while yin became associated in part with dark, black, cold, passivity, earth, and female.

Yang/yin theory states that life is not a dichotomy, but a dualism. A dichotomy is when the apparent opposites in nature, such as good and evil, beauty and ugliness, exist independently from each other. A dualism is an interdependent relationship between apparent opposites, i.e. one only calls something "good" by contrasting it with what they call "evil," and vice versa. One cannot exist without the other. We make the distinction between day (yang) and night (yin), yet we cannot have one without the other. One cannot be alive (yang) without dying and one cannot die (yin) without having been alive. Therefore yang/yin theory is a simple, basic way of observing and understanding change. However, this theory is relative to the sphere of influence one is discussing. Day is yang, night is yin, summer is yang, winter is yin, but day (yang) cannot be compared to winter (yin) as they are not in the same sphere of influence.

Everything that exists can be understood as an expression of the polarity of yang and yin. Some other yang/yin correspondences are as follows:

Yang 阳	Yin 阴
Above	Below
Day	Night
Summer	Winter
Fire	Water
External	Internal
Excess	Deficient
Function	Substance

b. Wǔ Xíng - the Five Phase Theory

From the dualism of yang/yin theory developed the Wǔ Xíng 五
行 or Five Phase theory. The change between the two fundamental
principles of yang and yin is now extrapolated to five interdependent
principles which promote and restrain each other as a means of
maintaining homeostasis, balance. The Five Phases correlate to many
aspects of life, yet are most often spoken of in terms of the five
elements; wood, fire, earth, metal, and water. Each of the Five Phases
generates or promotes the one immediately following it. Within wood
is the energy of fire, so wood is said to generate fire. Fire consumes
wood, turns it to ash, so fire is said to generate earth (ash). Within the
earth is found metals, so earth generates metal. In ancient China,
mirrors were made of polished metal, and in the morning, the mirror
would be covered in water (what we know as condensation), so metal
was said to generate water (also, when metal is heated it becomes
liquid). Water nurtures plant growth, so water generates wood, and the
cycle repeats. These are the five phases of change that all things are
said to proceed through.

Each phase also controls or restrains the second one following it;
wood controls earth, fire controls metal, earth controls water, metal
controls wood, and water controls fire. The generating and controlling
cycles are what maintains balance between the Five Phases. For
example, wood generates fire so fire can grow but water controls fire

so it doesn't become too strong. Water generates wood, yet metal keeps wood under control. This applies to all five phases. A failure of one or more of these cycles leads to imbalance and disharmony in nature and in humans.

There are two ways of diagraming the Five Phases. The first diagram is the most well-known and shows the generating cycle as circular and the controlling cycle as a five pointed star (wood generates fire and water controls fire, etc.). The second diagram is the cosmological arrangement.

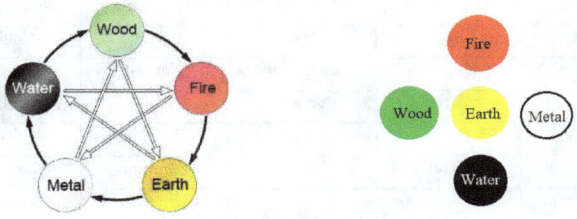

The cosmological arrangement appears in the oldest written mention of the Five Phases. It lists them as the north – 1, the south – 2, the east – 3, the west – 4, and the center – 5. North is water, south is fire, east is wood, west is metal, and earth is the center. The Chinese compass has north at the bottom and south at the top, hence 1 – north, 2 – south, etc. Five being the center also becomes what is referred to as the completion number. When the completion number 5 is added to 1 through 5, it makes 6 through 10. The numbers 1 through 5 are said to be representative of the energy of heaven and 6 through 10 the energy of earth. In the cosmological arrangement, wood/east and fire/south are considered yang (yang rises, wood floats, fire flares upward) and metal/west and water/north are considered yin (yin descends, metal sinks, water flows down). Earth, being the center, is yang and yin in balance, and represents the transformation between each seasonal element.

Some of the basic correlations of the Five Phases are as follows:

	Fire	Earth	Metal	Water	Wood
Direction	South	Center	West	North	East
Season	Summer May - June	Last month of season	Autumn Aug - Sept	Winter Nov - Dec	Spring Feb - Mar
Climate	Heat	Damp	Dry	Cold	Wind
Process	Growth	Transformation	Harvest	Storage	Birth
Color	Red	Yellow	White	Indigo Blue	Green
Taste	Bitter	Sweet	Pungent	Salty	Sour
Yin Organ	Heart	Spleen	Lung	Kidney	Liver
Yang Organ	Small Intestine	Stomach	Large Intestine	Bladder	Gallbladder
Opening	Tongue	Mouth	Nose	Ears	Eyes
Tissue	Vessels	Muscles	Skin	Bones	Sinews
Emotion	Joy	Pensiveness	Sadness	Fear	Anger
Sound	Laughing	Singing	Crying	Groaning	Shouting

c. The Hé Tú 河图, the Luò Shū 洛书, and the Nine Palaces (Jiǔ Gōng Tú) 九宫

According to legend, Fú Xī, the first of the three legendary emperors of pre-historic China (3rd millennium BCE), once saw a dragon-horse (lóng mǎ 龙马) rise out of the Yellow River with a distinct pattern on its back. This image is known as the Hé Tú or River

Diagram. This diagram became the basis for the first attempt at notating the concept of yang and yin, as well as the order of the Wu Xing cosmological arrangement.

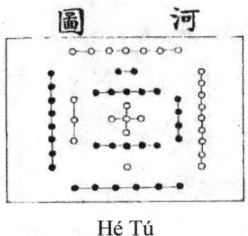

Hé Tú

As previously mentioned, yang is associated with light and white, yin with dark and black. Hence, the white dots in the Hé Tú, which are the odd numbers (1, 3, 5, 7, 9) are considered yang and the black dots, which are the even numbers (2, 4, 6, 8, 10) are considered yin. In Chinese medicine, performing a technique an odd number of times is considered yang and tonifying, while performing a technique an even number of times is considered yin and sedating.

Centuries after Fú Xī, pre-historic China was inundated by a great flood. No one could tame the floods until a man named Yǔ was given the task. He traveled the countryside for 13 years, dredging canals and redirecting rivers, and eventually the flood waters receded. He is known as Dà Yǔ 大禹 or Yu the Great, and became the third "sage king" after the Yellow Emperor, and the ruler of the first dynasty, the Xià (c. 2000 BCE).[4] During this momentous effort, Yǔ is said to have witnessed a dragon-turtle (lóng guī 龙龟) rise out of the Luò River with a pattern on its back similar to the Hé Tú. This image is known as the Luò Shū or Luò River Scroll.

Again, the white dots are the odd/yang numbers and the black dots are the even/yin numbers. The white dots are in the cardinal directions and the center, and the black dots are in the intercardinal directions. The Luò Shū was the influence for the Jiǔ Gōng Tú or the Nine Palaces diagram, also known as the magic square.

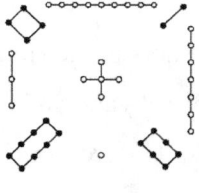

4	9	2
3	5	7
8	1	6

Luò Shū   Nine Palaces Diagram

The Nine Palaces diagram is pregnant with meaning in Chinese philosophy and medicine. Each square represents an external body part, an internal organ, the elements of the Wǔ Xíng, the trigrams of the Bā Guà, the Ten Celestial Stems, the Eight Extraordinary Vessels and their respective Confluent Points, as well as a direction, a season, and a month. My teacher told me if one understands the Nine Palaces, then one will know all there is to know about Chinese medicine. This diagram also plays a crucial role in the acupuncture-chronotherapy that will be discussed later.

d. Bā Guà 八卦 The Eight Divine Trigrams

At the time Fú Xī saw the pattern on the dragon-horse (lóng mǎ), there was no written language. He devised a way of notating the concept of yang and yin in accordance to the white/odd number dots and the black/even number dots. The number one was presented by a single line _____ while the number two was represented by a broken line ___ ___ consisting of two parts. The "one" single line represents yang, while the "two" broken lines represent yin. He combined them in groups of three lines called a trigram. There are eight possible combinations of the solid and broken line in groups of three, and these are called the bā guà or eight divine trigrams.

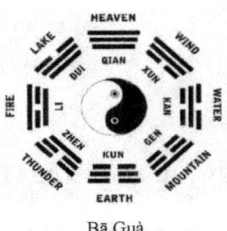

Bā Guà

A trigram is read from the bottom line up, and in this diagram, the inner most line in the circle is the bottom line. As such, beginning with zhèn – thunder in the bottom left corner and coming up the left side, yang increases until qián – heaven, which is pure yang. Then beginning with xùn – wind in the upper right corner and coming down the right side, yin increases until kūn – earth, which is pure yin. This is the pre-heaven arrangement, representing the energy cycle of heaven

15

and it inspired the creation of the yang yin tu (diagram), attributed to Lái Zhīdú (b. 1525 -d. 1604), shown here in the middle of the bā guà. It shows the rising of yang, which became the vast expanse of heaven, and the descending of yín, which became the dense earth. The yin tang tu is a simplified modern version of the ancient Wújí Tú 無極图 attributed to the Daoist sage Chén Tuán (b. 871 – d. 989).

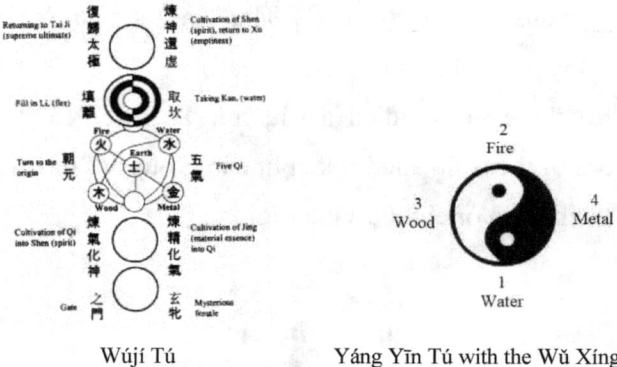

Wújí Tú   Yáng Yīn Tú with the Wǔ Xíng elements

e. Daoist Cosmology (yǔ zhòu xué 宇宙学)

The Daoist theory of the origin and development of the universe is represented by four symbols:

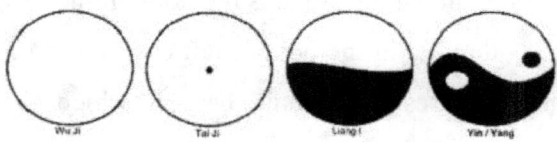

The empty circle represents Wújí 無極, literally "limitless, unbounded." It is the unrealized potential of all existence. It is

everything that exists in this world in an as yet unrealized state, the unmanifested potential for all existence.

The circle with a dot in the center represents Taiji 太极, the Supreme Ultimate, the unrealized potential of all existence becoming realized. Wuji is the substance (wù zhì 物质) of Taiji, Taiji is the function (gōng néng 功能) of Wuji. Wuji could be equated to the moment before the Big Bang or the moment before God created the universe, however one wants to conceptualize it. Taiji is the moment right after this event, when the potential started becoming realized, existence becoming manifest.

The half white, half black circle represents liang yi 两仪, literally two paths or two intentions. This is the manifesting potential of all existence beginning to diversify. Here Taiji is the substance, liang yi is the function. As the potential of existence becomes realized, two "paths" emerge. Liang yi is a concept we are faced with multiple times daily. To do or not to do, this vs that, etc. It's like coming to a fork in the road, but not yet choosing right or left. Both paths exist simultaneously. Cosmologically, it is the beginning of diversification.

Liang yi manifests as yin/yang 阴阳, the dualism of all existence represented by the yin yang tu (diagram). Here liang yi is the substance, yin/yang is the function. Once one makes the choice of this or that, chooses which fork in the road to follow, so to speak, yin/yang comes into being. This is similar to the concept of quantum observation; once an observation (choice) is made, it creates "reality."

Yin/yang become "all living things," wan wu 萬物. Here yin/yang is the substance, all living things are the function. This is the potential fully realized, the manifestation of the world of Ten Thousand Things in Daoism.

wújì huà tàijí	无际化太极	limitlessness transforms into Supreme Ultimate
tàijí huà shén	太极化神	Supreme Ultimate transforms into spirit
shén huà liǎngyí	神化两仪	spirit transforms into the two intentions
liǎngyí huà yīnyáng	仪化阴阳	the two intentions transforms into yin/yang
yīn yáng nǎi chéng wàn wù	阴阳乃成萬物	yin/yang become the ten thousand things

(It is interesting to note that this diagram can also represent the development of the human being. The empty circle represents the human oocyte, the circle with the dot the fertilized oocyte, the remainder of the circles human mitosis.)

f. Nèidān (Internal Alchemy) 内丹

Neidan or Internal Alchemy is the Daoist practice of self-cultivation. It encompasses a wide and varied assortment of traditions focusing on physical health, emotional well-being, and spiritual development. As humans are a microcosm of the universe, understanding how the Daoist concept of cosmology discussed above applies to human development is needed.

g. The Process of Manifestation or "Going Along"

The process of manifestation discussed above in relation to the universe is referred to in Daoist alchemy, as regards the human being, as "going along," (shùn huà 顺化, literally "continuing transformation"), i.e. the manifestation of the human being as a microcosm of the manifestation of the universe. As such:

xū huà shén	虚化神	emptiness transforms into spirit
shén huà qì	神化气	spirit transforms into energy
qì huà jīng	气化精	energy transforms into essence
jīng huà xíng	精乃形	essence transforms into form
xíng nǎi chéng rén	形乃成人	form then becomes the human being

In the Cantong Qi 参同契 (the Seal of the Unity of the Three), the oldest Daoist alchemical text, it states, "From the coagulation of the spirit the corporeal frame is formed. This is how all beings come to be." [5] This is another way of expressing the above process, that "all living things" begin on the spiritual or energetic level and manifest lastly on the physical level. Even the Law of Physics states that all matter is energy in various densities, and that energy cannot be created or destroyed, only altered.

As we "go along" with the natural process, we come into being in this world, we develop, age, and eventually the physical body dies. We begin in a pure state of primordial energy and devolve into the temporal state of conditioned existence.

"So it is that one encounters obscurity and shame, flowing along with the waves of life and death, sunk continually in the sea of suffering, having eternally lost the true Tao." [6]

h. Primordial vs Temporal

A very important distinction in Daoist alchemy is the concept of the primordial and the temporal. The primordial is the natural state of existence without bias or discrimination. In the primordial state, there is no distinction between essence and life, mind and body. Life is perceived "as-it-is," without subjective bias. We are born with this primordial state of pure consciousness. This is evidenced by observing an infant in the first years of life. They have no preconceived notions of existence, only a basic awareness of the moment "as-it-is," i.e. of being hungry, tired, cold, content, etc. Mind and body are one in the moment.

The temporal is that which relates to worldly affairs and the passage of time. Over time we become conditioned by our experiences, our physical interaction within this existence. As the years pass, we become more self-aware, me vs. not-me, and develop conceptual ideas about our surroundings and our place in it based on these experiences. This leads us to developing feelings, attitudes, and biases about life.

We humans are conscious beings. In the primordial state, our consciousness makes no distinction between mind and body.

Experiences are "as-they-are." Over time our consciousness has perceptions of our surroundings. We then make distinctions about our perceptions based primarily upon what we deem to be pleasant or unpleasant. Once a distinction is made, we give the perception an identity. This identity then becomes our subjective reality and creates an emotional response. Distinctions made based upon emotional feelings become the basis for our desires. Desire and seeking affect the mind and our ability to see the world clearly. This leads to a feeling of distress and worry over what we think we want and whether we can achieve it or not. Worry brings suffering to the body and mind, eventually separating our essence from life. Our body and mind, spirit and energy, once unified, are no longer one. Experiences now are as we perceive them, not necessarily as they truly are.

i. The Cultivation of Essence and Life (xìng-mìng xué)

A central concept in Daoist neidan is the cultivation of xing-ming 性命学. Chinese words are sometimes difficult to accurately translate into English. They can have contextual variations in meaning. Xing is essence and is also seen as mind or spirit. Ming is life and is also seen as body or energy. Originally xing/ming, mind/body, spirit/energy, are united in the primordial state only to become separated by temporal conditioning, as discussed above. Working towards the reunification of life with essence, body with mind, energy with spirit, returns the individual to the unified primordial state, and this is the purpose of neidan.

Various techniques are described in the Daoist texts on how to reunite ming with xing. All of them involve "doing" (yǒuwéi 有为), because they involve active practices. Once the culmination of practice has been achieved, the adept having returned to the unified primordial state, active work is no longer required. This stage is referred to as "non-doing" (wúwéi 无为), because when this is achieved there is no longer anything to "do," no work to be done. There is just "being." There is nothing left for the adept to accomplish, as they have returned to the unified, primordial consciousness.

One way of understanding xing-ming is in relation to the Wu Xing, the Five Phases. The Primordial state is the Original Mind, pure consciousness, unpolluted by Temporal conditioning. In the Primordial state, the human psyche is an aggregate of five parts; Basic Essence, Basic Sense, Basic Spirit, Basic Vitality, and Basic Energy. These are referred to as the Five Bases. In the Temporal state they represent the five parts of the human soul; the Hún or ethereal soul, the Pò or corporeal soul, Shén or conscious mind, the Zhì or vitality, and the Yì or intent, respectively.

In accordance with the Wu Xing, in the Primordial state Essence (wood/Hún) gives rise to Conscious Knowledge (fire/Shén). Conscious Knowledge gives rise to True Intent (earth/Yì). True Intent give rise to

True Sense (metal/Pò). True Sense gives rise to Real Knowledge (water/Zhì). Real Knowledge then fosters Essence and the Primordial state grows stronger.

Within the Primordial state of the Five Bases are the Five Virtues; benevolence, justice, courtesy, knowledge, and truthfulness. They are necessary for social health and personal development. However, due to Temporal conditioning, as described above, the Five Virtues devolve into emotions and cravings known as the Five Thieves; joy, anger, sadness, happiness, and lust. Again, in accordance with the Wu Xing, emotions and cravings of the Five Thieves cause True Sense to become Feelings. Feelings overcome Real knowledge, producing Desire. Desire overcomes Essence, producing Temperament. Temperament overcomes Conscious Knowledge, producing Volatility. Volatility overcomes True Intentions, producing Arbitrary Intentions. Arbitrary Intentions overcome True Sense, producing Feelings, which in turn causes Real Knowledge to become Desire, which produces Temperament.

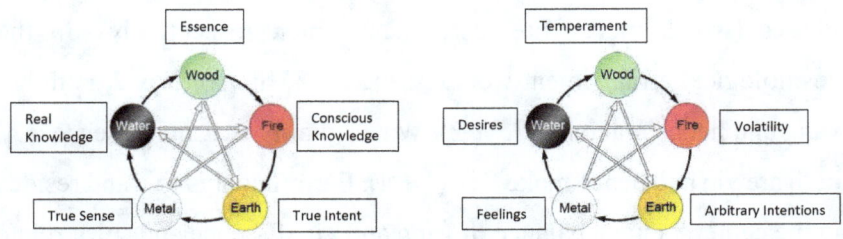

According to Quánzhēn 全真 (Complete Reality) Daoism, reverting from the conditioned Temporal state back to the Primordial state is the goal of internal alchemy. This is done by reversing the Generating cycle by overcoming Feelings so they revert to True Sense. True Sense then reverts Arbitrary Intentions to True Intent, True Intent reverts Volatility to Conscious Knowledge, Conscious Knowledge reverts Temperament to Essence, Essence reverts Desire to Real Knowledge, and Real Knowledge turns Feelings into True Sense.

j. The Concept of 3/5/1

Based on the cosmological arrangement of the Wu Xing we have the concept of 3/5/1. In the *Wuzhen pian* 悟真篇 or Comprehending Reality by Zhang Boduan it states, "Those who understand the three words "three, five one" have always been truly rare." [7] This refers to the three bases (basic essence, basic vitality, basic spirit discussed above), the five forces (essence, sense, spirit, intent, and vitality), and the one true energy. The five forces are also represented by the Five Phases (wood, metal, fire, earth, and water, respectively). In the cosmological arrangement wood/essence is 3, fire/spirit is 2, both are yang and hence make five (3 + 2). Water/vitality is 1, metal/sense is 4, both are yin and hence make five (1 + 4). Earth/intent is five and resides in the center, being a balance of yang and yin. Essence and spirit relate to the mind and make a set. Vitality and sense relate to the body and

24

make a set. Intent, in the center, is a set unto itself. These three sets, each adding up to five, are referred to as the three fives.

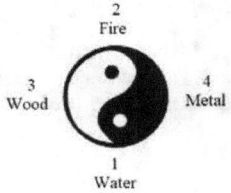

When the north 1 and the west 4 unite, the body is still and essence can be refined into breath (qi). When the east 3 and the south 2 unite, the mind is calm and breath can be refined into spirit. When the center five is focused, the intent does not waver and spirit can be refined back to emptiness. Body, mind, and intent (3) are still and calm, the center (5) is focused, and they revert to the true, primordial energy (1). This is referred to as "inverting the course" (nìxíng 逆行).

k. Inverting the Course (nìxíng 逆 行)

The goal of Daoist alchemy is "inverting the course" (nixing 逆行), that is, to reverse the process of manifestation, of "going along," and return to the primordial state of being (the Dao), which then promotes spiritual development and a long, healthy life. The first step is devoted to replenishing the Three Origins (sānyuán 三元); Original Essence (yuán jīng), Original Breath (yuán qì), and Original Spirit (yuán shén). This is "laying the foundation," the first stage in the

25

alchemical process. Only when the basic constituents of the body are replenished can the other stages of alchemical refinement be carried out properly.

"One reverts to the fundamental and returns to the root, enlightens one's mind, and sees one's Nature." [8] This process involves four stages:

yǎng xíng liàn jīng	養形鍊精	nourish form to refine into essence
jī jīng huà qì	积精化气	accumulate essence to transform into energy
liàn qì hé shén	鍊气合神	refine energy to merge with spirit
liàn shén huán xū	鍊神还虚	refine spirit to revert to emptiness

In the Qīng Jìng Jīng 清靜經 – The Classic of Clarity and Stillness, it says, "When people are able to be constantly clear and still, heaven and earth will be known and all will return (to the source)." [9]

l. The Three Treasures of Chinese Medicine

Having studied both Daoist philosophy for over 40 years and Chinese medicine for almost 20 years, the one defining constant between CCM and Daoist nèidān 內丹 (inner alchemy) is the theory of what is referred to as the Three Treasures in CCM and the Three Bases in nèidān. While understood in slightly different ways, the concept of these three is essential for the physical, mental, and spiritual well-being of the individual.

In Chinese medicine, jīng 精, qì 氣, and shén 神 are referred to as the Three Treasures and are the primary vital substances of the individual. The jing or essence is equated to an individual's inherited congenital make-up and is stored in the kidneys. It is further differentiated as pre-heaven essence and post-heaven essence. The pre-heaven essence is inherited from parents and ancestors and the post-heaven essence is acquired from lifestyle. Pre-heaven essence is finite; what you're born with is all you get. However, it can be augmented by post-heaven essence which is acquired through a proper lifestyle including diet, exercise, and balancing work with rest.

The energy or qi of the body is also derived in part from the post-heaven essence as it comes from the food and drink consumed and is formed in the spleen. The literal translation of qi means air, the same as the word prana in the yogic tradition and the word spiritus in Latin (from which we get the word spirit). They all literally mean air, but represent the animating factor, the vital life force, in all living things. This energy is vital to all the functions of the body including individual organ functions.

Spirit or shen is the least material aspect of the individual and constitutes cognition and mental function. According to Chinese medicine the mind is housed in the heart. Hence, the Three Treasures are housed in the three sections of the torso (pelvic, abdominal, thoracic) referred to as the sānjiāo 三焦 or triple heater. The lower jiao houses the kidneys, middle jiao the spleen, and upper jiao the heart.

The Three Treasures also reflect the Three Powers, which are Heaven (pure yang), Earth (pure yin), and Humans (both yang and yin). After yang and yin separated, with yang becoming the vast expanse of Heaven and yin the turbid dense Earth, they want to reconnect. The yang of Heaven descends to influence the yin of Earth, which rises in response, and we humans are the conduit through which this energetic cycle happens.

Part Two - Daoism and Acupuncture

a) Acupuncture

The basic theories of Chinese medicine are founded in Daoism (dào jiào), the indigenous, fundamental principle at the center of Chinese philosophical and spiritual thought. The central concepts of Daoism pre-date Chinese history. The ancient's desire to understand the world led them to observe and study the basic concept of existence, that of change. The fact that all things undergo change is the only thing in life that never changes. Understanding change, both in the physical world and within the human body, is the central concept of Daoist philosophy and Chinese medicine, both of which begin with observation (wáng 望 or looking – literally to gaze into the distance).

No one knows exactly how far back into antiquity the practice of acupuncture goes. The first needles were made of stone and were called biān 砭. Metal needles have been used since around 800 BCE. An archeological dig at Mǎwángduī of a Hàn dynasty tomb sealed in 168 BCE discovered acupuncture needles made of gold and silver, and written discussions of medical problem. All of the basic concepts of Chinese medicine, from theory to diagnostics to treatment protocols were firmly established by the Hàn dynasty (206 BCE–220 CE).

The oldest book on Chinese medicine is the Huáng Dì Nèi Jīng, the Yellow Emperor's Inner Classic, comprised of two books, the Sù Wěn (Plain Questions) which discusses theory and the Líng Shū

(Spiritual Pivot) which discusses acupuncture in particular. Although named after the Yellow Emperor (b. 2711 BCE - d. 2599 BCE), one of the three legendary emperors of ancient China, this book is now believed to have been composed during the Hàn dynasty. The version we have today was compiled by Wáng Bìng in 762 CE.

b) The Jīng Luò 经络 and the Zàng Fǔ 脏腑

The jīng luò are the channels (jīng) and collaterals (luò) that make up the energetic system that connects the body into an integrated whole. They are like the threads of a spider web, some larger, some smaller, but all are interconnected. There are twelve primary channels, each one associated with and named in accordance to one of twelve zàng fǔ, the twelve internal organs; Lung, Large Intestine, Stomach, Spleen, Heart, Small Intestine, Bladder, Kidney, Pericardium, San Jiao, Gallbladder, and Liver.

The theory of yin/yang is applied to the organs/channels with each having either a yin identity or a yang identity. This is based on the concept of yin being substance and internal, and yang being function and external (part 1, section A). The yin organs store the vital life substances and are considered internal. They are the Lungs, Spleen, Heart, Kidney, and Liver (the Pericardium is seen as a part of the Heart). The yang organs transport nutrients and waste (function) and are considered external. They are the Large Intestine, Stomach, Small

Intestine, Bladder, and Gallbladder (the San Jiao in this case is different from the three section of the body mentioned above and is an organ "with a name but no location." [10] The San Jiao "organ" is considered by many as the connective tissue, having no specific location as it is found throughout the body.)

Each of the primary channels have "points" along its pathway where the qi (energy) of the body can be accessed. The actual Chinese name for what we call an acupuncture point is xuè 穴, which means cave or cavity and is where the qi of the respective organs/channels can be accessed.

c) The 8 Extraordinary Vessels and the Confluent Points

The 8 Extraordinary Vessels (qí jīng bā mài 奇經八脈) are somewhat elusive and overlooked in modern acupuncture theory, in my opinion. According to Peter Deadman, et al, in "A Manual of Acupuncture," the standard text used in acupuncture schools, they are "reservoirs which are able to absorb excessive qi and blood from the primary channels." [11] They are also seen as part of the web which links the 12 primary channels, thus uniting the body into an integrative whole. This is a parochial and shallow view of an integral aspect of this amazing medicine.

First of all, we must ask why are they referred to as "extraordinary"? There are several reasons for this. They are not considered a part of the jīng-luò channel system, comprised of the 12 primary channels, the luò-connecting channels, the divergent channels, etc. They are not paired as internal-external couples the way the primary channels are. They are not paired as yīn-yáng couples the way the primary channels are. They are not connected to a specific internal organ (zàng fǔ) the way the primary channels are. Except for the Du and Ren, they do not have points of their own. But even more importantly, the Extraordinary Vessels are an expression of the underlying, primordial energetic matrix which is actually the basis for the remainder of the jīng-luò structure. As Charles Chase says, in his introduction to Lǐ Shí-Zhēn's "An Exposition on the Eight Extraordinary Vessels," "The eight extraordinary vessels are not bound to the primary vessels in the same way as the secondary vessels. Each extraordinary vessel exerts its own influence on every channel to one extent or another. Each exercises its regulatory effect on the entire body. They are the matrix that provides the gross structure for the rest of the channel system." [12]

In the first 2 – 3 weeks of mitosis there is no regulatory system; no organs, no blood vessels, no nerves, no bones, only cells communicating, dividing, and beginning to specialize. During gastrulation, the embryo folds creating what Western medicine calls the primitive streak, which is actually the chòng mài (thoroughfare vessel), the first energetic channel to develop in what will become the body. This becomes the mesoderm. Next the rèn mài (conception vessel - endoderm) and the dū mài (governing vessel - ectoderm) develop. These three are bound together by the dài mài (girdling vessel), the only horizontal channel in the body. The yīn qiào mài and yáng qiào mài (motility vessels) develop, allowing for the upward and downward flow of qi in the body and the yīn wéi mài and yáng wéi mài (linking vessels) develop, which link the internal and external flow of qi.

Each of the extraordinary vessels have a confluent point. A confluence, usually used in terms of bodies of water such as rivers, are where two or more things converge and come together. Where the Missouri river joins the Mississippi river is the confluent point of these two rivers. The confluent points are located on one of the primary channels and are where the extraordinary vessels converge with the primary channels. Again, the extraordinary vessels are the precursors to the primary channels and are the original energetic matrix of the body, and it is at these locations that the extraordinary vessels connect with and influence the primary channel system and hence, the zàng fǔ.

The extraordinary vessels, as well as the confluent points, are arranged in four pairs, and are paired yang with yang and yin with yin. This arrangement has been credited to Dou Han-Qing in the Yuan dynasty (1295). Dou claimed this knowledge was in a book written and given to him by a Daoist sage named Shao Shi, however the book has been lost to antiquity.

<u>Dou Han-Qing's Pairing of the Confluent Points</u>

Father	SP 4	Gōngsūn	communicates with the Chòng Mài
Mother	PC 6	Nèiguān	communicates with the Yīn Wéi Mài
Husband	SI 3	Hòu Xī	communicates with the Dū Mài
Wife	BL 62	Shēn Mài	communicates with the Yáng Qiāo Mài
Male	GB 41	Zú Lín Qì	communicates with the Dài Mài
Female	SJ 5	Wài Guān	communicates with the Yáng Wéi Mài
Host	LU 7	Liè Quē	communicates with the Rèn Mài
Guest	KD 6	Zhào Hǎi	communicates with the Yīn Qiāo Mài

The numbering system we have for the points, i.e. SP 4, PC 6, has only been around since the 1980's. We don't know why they are paired as they are, possibly having to do with their names, as in antiquity the names had something to do with either the location or function of the points. There are, however, some interesting correlations between these channels.

The first pair we look at is the Du and Yang Qiao. The Du is a yang channel, is external, and the Du channel flows up the center line of the back of the body. The Confluent point is SI 3 and the Small Intestine channel flows up from the hand to the face. The Yang Qiao is a yang channel, is external, and the flow of qi is down the lateral aspect of the body. The Confluent point is BL 62 and the Bladder channel flows down the posterior-lateral aspect of the body from the face to the foot.

Next is the Ren and Yin Qiao. The Ren is a yin channel, is internal, and the Ren channel flows down the center line of the front of the body. The Confluent point is Lu 7 and the Lung channel flows down the medial aspect of the arm from the chest to the hand. The Yin Qiao is a yin channel, is internal, and the Yin Qiao flows up the medial aspect of the legs. The Confluent point is KD 6 and the Kidney channel flows up the medial aspect of the legs from the foot to the chest.

The Dai is a yang channel, is external, and the Dai channel encircles the body at the waist, the only horizontal channel in the body. The Confluent point is SJ 5 and the San Jiao channel flows up the lateral aspect of the arms from the hand to the face. The San Jiao, being the organ "with a name but no location," is recognized in many circles as the fascia, the connective tissue, and hence it also encompasses the entire body. As the Dai encircles the body horizontally, so does the San Jiao vertically. The Yang Wei is a yang channel, is external, and the Yang Wei flows down the lateral aspect of the body. The Confluent point is GB 41 and the Gallbladder channel flows down The lateral aspect of the body from the face to the foot.

The Chong is a yin channel, is internal, and the Chong flows up the center of the body. The Confluent point is SP 4 and the Spleen channel flows up the medial aspect of the legs from the foot to the chest.

The Yin Wei is a yin channel, is internal, and the Yin Wei flows down the anterior-medial aspect of the body. The Confluent point is PC 6 and the Pericardium channel flows down the medial aspect of the arms from the chest to the hand.

With this pairing, we see the flow of qi in the Extraordinary Vessels is a continuous movement of upward and downward, inward and outward cycles.

d) The Gān Zhī, the 10 Celestial Stems, and the 12 Branches

According to legend, Huáng Dì, the Yellow Emperor, asked his advisor, the Daoist sage Dà Rǎo Shì, to devise a way to mark the passage of time. Dà Rǎo Shì observed the cycles of heaven and earth, the passage of the seasons, and devised the Gān Zhī 干支, the sexagenarian cycle, or cycle of 60. This applies to the four pillars of time in the Chinese calendar; years, months, days, and hours. For the cycles of heaven, he devised the Ten Celestial Stems (Shí Tiāngān 十天干) and for the cycles of earth, the Twelve Terrestrial Branches (Shí Èr Zhī 十二枝). The Ten Stems are each associated with one of the elements of the Five Phases, each stem having either a yang or yin nature. The Twelve Branches represent the twelve animals of the Chinese zodiac, each also having either a yang or yin nature.

The Stems and Branches are as follows:

The 10 Celestial Stems					The 12 Terrestrial Branches			
S1	Jiǎ	yang	wood		B1	Zǐ	Rat	yang
S2	Yǐ	yin	wood		B2	Chǒu	Ox	yin
S3	Bǐng	yang	fire		B3	Yín	Tiger	yang
S4	Dīng	yin	fire		B4	Mǎo	Rabbit	yin
S5	Wù	yang	earth		B5	Chén	Dragon	yang
S6	Jǐ	yin	earth		B6	Sì	Snake	yin
S7	Gēng	yang	metal		B7	Wǔ	Horse	yang
S8	Xīn	yin	metal		B8	Wèi	Sheep	yin
S9	Rén	yang	water		B9	Shēn	Monkey	yang
S10	Guǐ	yin	water		B10	Yǒu	Rooster	yin
					B11	Xū	Dog	yang
					B12	Hài	Pig	yin

For simplicity sake, the stems are abbreviated as S1, S2, S3, etc., and the branches as B1, B2, B3, etc. They begin the correlation with S1 aligned with B1, then S2 with B2, and so on. However, there are only ten stems vs twelve branches, so after S10 aligns with B10, the stems revert to S1 but the branches continue to B11, then S2 and B12. Because of this, S1 and B1 will not realign again until after the sixtieth pairing when S10 aligns with B12 and the cycle will begin again.

B1	B2	B3	B4	B5	B6	B7	B8	B9	B10	B11	B12
S1B1	S2B2	S3B3	S4B4	S5B5	S6B6	S7B7	S8B8	S9B9	S10B10	S1B11	S2B12
S3B1	S4B2	S5B3	S6B4	S7B5	S8B6	S9B7	S10B8	S1B9	S2B10	S3B11	S4B12
S5B1	S6B2	S7B3	S8B4	S9B5	S10B6	S1B7	S2B8	S3B9	S4B10	S5B11	S6B12
S7B1	S8B2	S9B3	S10B4	S1B5	S2B6	S3B7	S4B8	S5B9	S6B10	S7B11	S8B12
S9B1	S10B2	S1B3	S2B4	S3B5	S4B6	S5B7	S6B8	S7B9	S8B10	S9B11	S10B12

The Gān Zhī or Sexagenarian Cycle of Sixty

Every year will be a different zodiac animal according to the progression of the Twelve Branches. Because of the offset of Ten Stems to Twelve Branches, every year will be a different element of the Five Phases in accordance to the Generating cycle. As an example, if you were born in 1984, that was an S1 B1 year or the year of the yang wood rat (see tables above). 1985 was an S2B2 year or the year of the yin wood ox. 1986 was an S3B3 year or yang fire tiger, 1987 was an S4B4 or yin fire rabbit, and so on. Every twelve years, an animal will repeat, however it will be a different element in accordance to the generating cycle of the wŭ xíng. 1984 was the wood rat, 1996 the fire rat, 2008 the earth rat, 2020 was the metal rat, 2032 will be the water rat, and 2044 will be the next time the year will be the wood rat, sixty years after 1984. The element/animal of the year you were born will not repeat until the year you turn 60.

The sexagenarian cycle also applies to days and hours. Each two hour time period is associated with a branch as follows:

Hour	Branch	Day Stem	Day Stem	Day Stem	Day Stem	Day Stem
23 to 1	B1 Zǐ	S1 Jiǎ	S3 Bǐng	S5 Wù	S7 Gēng	S9 Rén
1 to 3	B2 Chǒu	S2 Yǐ	S4 Dīng	S6 Jǐ	S8 Xīn	S10 Guǐ
3 to 5	B3 Yín	S3 Bǐng	S5 Wù	S7 Gēng	S9 Rén	S1 Jiǎ
5 to 7	B4 Mǎo	S4 Dīng	S6 Jǐ	S8 Xīn	S10 Guǐ	S2 Yǐ
7 to 9	B5 Chén	S5 Wù	S7 Gēng	S9 Rén	S1 Jiǎ	S3 Bǐng
9 to 11	B6 Sì	S6 Jǐ	S8 Xīn	S10 Guǐ	S2 Yǐ	S4 Dīng
11 to 13	B7 Wǔ	S7 Gēng	S9 Rén	S1 Jiǎ	S3 Bǐng	S5 Wù
13 to 15	B8 Wèi	S8 Xīn	S10 Guǐ	S2 Yǐ	S4 Dīng	S6 Jǐ
15 to 17	B9 Shēn	S9 Rén	S1 Jiǎ	S3 Bǐng	S5 Wù	S7 Gēng
17 to 19	B10 Yǒu	S10 Guǐ	S2 Yǐ	S4 Dīng	S6 Jǐ	S8 Xīn
19 to 21	B11 Xū	S1 Jiǎ	S3 Bǐng	S5 Wù	S7 Gēng	S9 Rén
21 to 23	B12 Hài	S2 Yǐ	S4 Dīng	S6 Jǐ	S8 Xīn	S10 Guǐ

The first two columns show the circadian clock two-hour times periods and the twelve branches associated with them. The remaining five columns show the ten stems in succession juxtaposed against the branches. This, again, results in a sixty hour cycle beginning with the pairing of S1B1 and ending with the pairing of S10B12, and the cycle begins again.

Once the stem and branch of a given day has been determined, it is easy to follow the progression on the sixty day, sexagenarian cycle. How to calculate the stem and branch of a day is covered in my book on the Ling Gui Ba Fa 灵龟八法, or Eight Methods of the Sacred Turtle, however, to make it easier for the practitioner to utilize the Ling Gui Ba Fa, without having to go through the complicated steps of calculating the "open" point, I've included a simple chart which can be used very easily to determine the points to be used on any day. (See Appendix A and B below)

e) The Sexagenarian Cycle and Acupuncture

Applying the cycle of sixty to treatment protocols is a form of chronotherapy. Chronotherapy involves specific treatments done at specific times. In Classical Chinese Medicine, this includes herbal remedies as well as acupuncture. The first reference we have to chronotherapy was by Zhang Zhongjing, in his seminal work *Shan Han Lun* (Treatise on Cold Disease), in which he mentions that illnesses tend to naturally improve during specific time periods of the day and the importance of prescribing herbal formulas to be ingested at those times to enhance the body's ability to heal. [13]

Chrono-acupuncture involves needling specific acupoints at certain times to have the best possible effect on the body. The first mention of chrono-acupuncture was by He Rou-You, in the Song dynasty (960 -1279 CE). There are several acupuncture chronotherapies, but some stand out from the rest, both in theory and in efficacy. One in particular is the Ling Gui Ba Fa 灵龟八法, or Eight Methods of the Sacred Turtle, mentioned above, an ancient Daoist acupuncture protocol first written about in great detail by Yang Jizhou in *"Great Compendium of Acupuncture and Moxibustion"* (*Zhen Jiu Da Cheng*), published in 1601.[14] This technique utilizes the Confluent Points of the Extraordinary Vessels combined with the theory of the 10 Celestial Stems and the 12 Terrestrial Branches, and the Nine Palaces. During each of the two-hour periods of the 24-hour day, one of the the 8 Confluent Points is "open" or active and is used with its coupled point. The two points (4 needles) can be used alone or with other points.

f) The Ling Gui Ba Fa Technique

When using the Ling Gui Ba Fa technique, the Confluent point that is "open" is considered the "ruling point" and its coupled point should also be selected. There are three ways this treatment can be applied: by appointed time, by random time, or by random time with other points, all three tapping into the primordial energetic matrix of the body. The last two are more conducive to the modern clinic as explained below.

1. Application at Appointed Times

When the patient calls to schedule an appointment, the confluent point which treats the respective condition is determined as well as the two-hour period in which the point will be open. For instance, if the patient complains of abdominal pain and diarrhea, the appropriate point(s) to use would be SP 4 and PC 6. The treatment would be scheduled on the day when SP 4 is the open point. However, this method is not always relevant to the modern clinic as the hours of operation may not facilitate this way of scheduling. Perhaps the respective point won't be open for several days or at an inconvenient time, such as 3:00 – 5:00 AM. The patient would not want to wait or come at that time.

2) Application at Random Times

This is the easiest way to use the Ling Gui Ba Fa. Regardless of the patient's chief complaint and which point would be most effective as described above, the open point at the time of the patient's appointment is to be used. As always, its coupled point is to also be used. For example, if the patient's appointment is on an S3B3 Bing Yin day between the hours of 1:00 and 3:00 PM, the open point is GB 41, the primary point, and should be paired with its coupled point, SJ 5 (see Appendix B, Open Point Table). This can be a stand-alone treatment, or more effectively, used as described next.

3) Application at Random Times with Other Points

This is done using the open Confluent point(s) first and then adding systemic points to reinforce the energetic effect of the Confluent points or adding empirical points to the Confluent point treatment. In either case, the number of needles used can and should be kept to a minimum. For example, the patient's chief complaint is low back pain. Use the "open" point first, then its coupled point, adding BL 23, BL 40, and KD 3. Or if the patient complains of shoulder pain, use the "open" point first followed by its coupled point, then add ST 38, the empirical point for shoulder pain.

The Ling Gui Ba Fa technique can also be applied to the following treatments described below. Use the "open" point first, followed by its coupled point, then one of the following treatments.

g) Neidan Treatments

In accordance with the concepts of Daoist internal alchemy described previously, I have developed some protocols which I use to treat patients on the energetic/spiritual level more so than on the physical level, although these treatments do elicit a physical response.

Besides the flow of qi up the Du and down the Ren, the qi also flows up the left and down the right. This is in accordance to the Wu Xing where the Liver/wood rises on the left and the Lung/metal descends on the right. Needling the right side first prepares the body for the acceptance of the qi from the left. In pulling the needles, pull the left first, then the right, allowing this flow to continue.

In "Classical Chinese Medicine" by Liu Lihong, he states, "spirit is primary to form," and "the higher level physician works to protect this aspect" (the spirit). [15] Treating the physical body results in a physical response, whereas treating the patient energetically will not only result in a physical response, but also in a psycho-emotional response. And the majority of illness these days is of a psycho-emotional origin.

In the Qīng Jìng Jīng 清靜經 – The Classic of Clarity and Stillness, it says that "worry brings suffering to the body and mind" and that a person then becomes "submerged in the ocean of misery."[16] Emotional disturbance, which is the result of the separation of xing/essence from ming/life as discussed above, is the root of most physical ailments. Look at the word disease. Dis- is the prefix meaning not, so disease is not being at ease. Even Western medicine has related stress to the top killers in this country including heart disease, cancer, respiratory ailments, stroke, accidents, and suicide.

1. 3/5/1 Treatment

This treatment is very effective for individuals who are suffering the stressors of daily life. They become fragmented, often not knowing where to turn or what to do to get back to a calm, centered life. For these patients I use the following treatment based on the concept of 3/5/1 mentioned above. "Three" represents of the jing (essence), qi (energy), and shen (spirit). "Five" represents the Five Forces or the Five Phases (wood, fire, earth, metal, water), each one also associated with one of the zang organs as well as the Wǔ Shèn (Five Spirits). "One" is the one true, primordial energy. There is a saying in neidan, "Refining Essence into Qi depends on the body not moving. Refining Qi into Spirit depends on the Mind not moving. Refining Spirit into Emptiness depends on the intent not moving." [17]

When the body is still the jing is refined into qi. When the mind is calm the qi is merges with shen. When the intent is focused the shen reverts to emptiness, and one unites with the true, primordial energy. Stilling the body is the north 1 (water/zhi) and the west 4 (metal/po) joining. Since the body is yin, this is done by needling the respective back-shu points, first BL 23 (kidney/zhi) and then BL 13 (lung/po), alternating right side first, then left (i.e., R-BL 23, L-BL 23, R-BL 13, L-BL 13). Calming the mind is the east 3 (wood/hun) and the south 2 (fire/shen) joining. Since the mind is yang, this is done by needling the respective spirit points, first BL 47 (liver/hun) and then BL 44 (heart/shen), again right side first. The intent not wavering is the center 5 (earth/yi). Since the center/intent is yin and yang in harmony, needle both the spirit point and the back-shu point, first BL 49 and then BL 20 (both spleen/yi), right, then left. In accordance to the theory of qi circulation in the Líng Shū (see section H below), allow the patient to rest for 30 minutes.

So the insertion order, needling right then left, is BL 23, BL 13, BL 47, BL 44, BL 49, BL 20. When pulling the needles, reverse the insertion order, pulling the left first, then the right; BL 20, BL 49, BL 44, BL 47, BL 13, and BL 23, returning shen from emptiness, reverting shen to qi, and finally qi to jing. (12 needles)

2) Combining the 3/5/1 with the Sān Guān 三關

For a very strong effective treatment, first use the 3/5/1 treatment described above, then open the San Guan as described below. As mentioned earlier, there are three energetic gates which correspond to the Three Bases that are to be opened in the practice of neidan. They are the wěilú guān (caudal funnel or sacral gate), jiājǐ guān (spinal handle gate), and the yúzhèn guān (jade pillow gate). Opening these three gates is part of the hé chē or River Chariot meditation which involves opening the Du and Ren channels to circulate qi continuously and facilitate health and well-being. Caution should be exercised initially in opening these gates as any repressed psycho-emotional issues the patient has not dealt with may be released.

To open the Three Gates, first needle Yùtián (jade field), on the midline of the sacrum below the fourth sacral foramen, to open the wěilǘ guān (caudal funnel gate). Next needle Du 11 Shén Dào (spirit path) at T5 directly behind the heart to open the jiājǐ guān (spinal handle gate). Lastly needle Du 17 Nǎohù (brain's door) above the external occipital protuberance to open the yúzhěn guān (jade pillow gate). Again, in accordance to the theory of qi circulation in the Líng Shū, allow the patient to rest for 30 minutes, then pull the needles in the reverse order, closing the yúzhěn guān, the jiājǐ guān, the wěilǘ guān, and then BL 20, BL 49, BL 47, BL 44, BL 13, and BL 23. (15 needles)

3) Hé Chē 河车 (The River Chariot)

This treatment is based on the River Chariot meditation, also known as the Waterwheel, the Micro-Cosmic Orbit, or the Small Heavenly Circuit (xiǎo zhōu tiān 小周天). This involves bringing the yin qi of earth up the Du channel, which joins with the yang qi of heaven in the center of the brain (níwán or muddy pellet) before descending down the Ren. Continuously circulating the qi in this way leads to spiritual development and physical health. According to Zhang Boduan, the founder of the southern school of Quánzhēn 全

真 (Complete Reality) Daoism, before one can open the Du, Ren, and Chong, one must first open the Yin Qiao. [18]

To open this circulation of qi, needle the confluent points of the respective Extraordinary Vessels as follows. Always needle the right side first. Begin by needling KD 6 to open the Yin Qiao, allowing the yin qi of the earth to enter the legs, flowing to the perineum at Ren 1, also known as díhù 地戶, earth's door, where the yin qi enters the body. Then needle SI 3 to open the Du, allowing the qi to rise up the back. Next, open the Three Gates (Sān Guān) as described above, then needle DU 20, also known as tiānmén 天門 (heaven's gate) to allow the yang qi of heaven to descend into the brain where it meets with the yin qi of earth. Next needle LU 7 to open the Ren allowing the qi to descend the front of the body, returning to díhù. Pull the needles in the same order as insertion, left side first. (10 needles)

A variation on this treatment is based on the Large Heavenly Circuit (dà zhōu tiān 大周天). After completing the above treatment, add SP 4 to open the Chong, bringing the qi up the center line to the chest, then PC 6 to open the Yin Wei, allowing the qi to descend the medial arm. Since PC 6 is also the Luo-Connecting point of the Pericardium, connecting the PC to the San Jiao, and SJ 5 is both the confluent point of the Yang Wei and the Luo-Connecting point connecting the SJ to the PC, and these points are on the medial and lateral aspects of the forearms across from each other, it is not necessary to needle SJ 5. Finally, needle BL 62 to open the Yang Qiao, allowing the qi to flow back down to the feet. In this way, the circulation of qi is up the medial legs to the perineum, up the posterior body to the head, down the anterior body to the perineum, up the center of the body to the chest, down the medial arms to the hands, up the lateral arms to the head, and down the lateral legs to the feet, then repeating. (16 needles). Again, pull the needles in the same order as insertion, left side first.

h) The Circulation of Qi in the Body According to the Ling Shu [19]

The ancient Chinese used a water clock, what the Greeks called a Clepsydra, to tell time. The Chinese water clock divided the 24-hour day into 50 equal segments, theoretically 25 daytime segments and 25 nighttime segments. In the *Ling Shu* or Spiritual Pivot, the second book in the *Huang Di Nei Jing* or Yellow Emperor's Inner Classic, it says, on Scroll 2, Chapter 5 – Roots and Ends:

"Within one day and one night, the nourishing qi circulates 50 times and nourishes the essence of the 5 viscera."

Thus, the ancient sages believed that the qi circulated one complete time during each of the 50 segments. Current belief is that an acupuncture treatment should last 15-20 minutes. My teacher said no longer than 30 minutes. But what is the optimal length for an acupuncture treatment? How long is a single segment of qi flow according to the *Ling Shu*?

Start by multiplying 24 hours by 60 minutes in each hour. This equals a total of 1440 minutes in a 24-hour period. Next divide 1440 minutes by 50 segments of the day; this equals 28.8 minutes for each segment. According to this theory, the qi cycles every 28.8 minutes, so the optimum length of a treatment should be 29 minutes. But can this be verified?

In Scroll 4, Chapter 17 – The Limits of the Channels, the *Ling Shu* states:

"The yang channels of the hand are 5 chi each. The yin channels of the hand are 3 chi 5 cun each. The yang channels of the foot are 8 chi each.

The yin channels of the foot are 6 chi 5 cun each. The qiao channels are 7 chi 5 cun each. The Du and Ren channels are 4 chi 5 cun each."

There are 10 cun in 1 chi, so the measurements by cun are:

Yang channels of the hand   50 cun x 6 channels = 300 cun or 30 chi
Yin channels of the hand   35 cun x 6 channels = 210 cun or 21 chi
Yang channels of the foot   80 cun x 6 channels = 480 cun or 48 chi
Yin channels of the foot   65 cun x 6 channels = 390 cun or 39 chi
Qiao channels   75 cun x 2 channels = 150 cun or 15 chi
<u>Du and Ren channels   45 cun x 2 channels =   90 cun or   9 chi</u>
Total   1620 cun or 162 chi

So the qi travels 162 chi in 1 cycle.

In Scroll 4, Chapter 15 – The 50 Regulators, it states:

"For one complete breath there is a traveling motion of the qi of 6 cun."

"In 270 breaths, the qi travels 162 chi. The qi travels, crosses and penetrates in the center within one revolution through the body."

"In 13,500 breaths, the qi travels the 50 regulators, 50 revolutions through the body."

"Consequently, 50 revolutions is a completion."

"Within the total movement is 810 times 10 chi." (81,000 cun)

This can be further calculated as follows:

270 breaths divided by 28.8 minutes = 9.4 breaths per minute

13,500 breaths divided by 270 breaths = 50 cycles

81,000 cun divided by 50 cycles = 1620 cun (162 chi) per cycle

The following calculations can now be applied:

Length of the channel divided by 162 = % of the total that qi travels in 1 revolution

270 breaths multiplied by the % traveled = # of breaths per channel per 1 revolution

28.8 minutes multiplied by the % traveled = # of minutes of qi travel through each channel per 1 revolution

As such we can understand the flow of qi through the channels as follows:

Yang channels of the hand	30 chi	50 breaths	5.3 minutes	18.5%
Yin channels of the hand	21 chi	35 breaths	3.7 minutes	13.0%
Yang channels of the foot	48 chi	80 breaths	8.5 minutes	29.6%
Yin channels of the foot	39 chi	65 breaths	7.0 minutes	24.0%
Qiao channels	15 chi	25 breaths	2.7 minutes	9.3%
Du and Ren channels	9 chi	15 breaths	1.6 minutes	5.6%
Total	162 chi	270 breaths	28.8 minutes	100%

Therefore, the qi does make a complete circulation of the body during each of the 50 cycles of the day in 28.8 minutes. Based on this calculation from the *Ling Shu*, the optimal time for an acupuncture treatment is a minimum of 29 minutes.

Appendix A: Treating with Ling Gui Ba Fa

Using the following chart, find the current date and the corresponding Stem and Branch of that day. Each section shows ten days. The top line shows the first day of each 60 day cycle. The chart can be updated using the Stem and Branch of the year (lines 39 -60). Once the Stem and Branch of the day has been determined, use the next chart to determine Confluent point that is "open."

	Year		Day							
1 Jia Zi		1/11/22	3/12/22	5/11/22	7/10/22	9/8/22	11/7/22	1/6/23	3/7/23
2 Yi Chou									
3 Bing Yin									
4 Ding Mao									
5 Wu Chen									
6 Ji Si									
7 Geng Wu									
8 Xin Wei									
9 Ren Shen									
10 Gui You									
11 Jia Xu		1/21/22	3/22/22	5/21/22	7/20/22	9/18/22	11/17/22	1/16/23	3/17/23
12 Yi Hai									
13 Bing Zi									
14 Ding Chou									
15 Wu Yin									
16 Ji Mao									
17 Geng Chen								CNY	
18 Xin Si									
19 Ren Wu									
20 Gui Wei									
21 Jia Shen		1/31/22	4/1/22	5/31/22	7/30/22	9/28/22	11/27/22	1/26/23	3/27/23
22 Yi You									
23 Bing Xu									
24 Ding Hai									
25 Wu Zi									
26 Ji Chou									
27 Geng Yin									
28 Xin Mao									
29 Ren Chen									
30 Gui Si									

31 Jia Wu		2/10/22	4/11/22	6/10/22	8/9/22	10/8/22	12/7/22	2/5/23	4/6/23
32 Yi Wei									
33 Bing Shen									
34 Ding You									
35 Wu Xu									
36 Ji Hai									
37 Geng Zi									
38 Xin Chou									
39 Ren Yin	2022								
40 Gui Mao	2023								
41 Jia Chen	2024	2/20/22	4/21/22	6/20/22	8/19/22	10/18/22	12/17/22	2/15/23	4/16/23
42 Yi Si	2025								
43 Bing Wu	2026								
44 Ding Wei	2027								
45 Wu Shen	2028								
46 Ji You	2029								
47 Geng Xu	2030								
48 Xin Hai	2031								
49 Ren Zi	2032								
50 Gui Chou	2033								
51 Jia Yin	2034	3/2/22	5/1/22	6/30/22	8/29/22	10/28/22	12/27/22	2/25/23	4/26/23
52 Yi Mao	2035								
53 Bing Chen	2036								
54 Ding Si	2037								
55 Wu Wu	2038								
56 Ji Wei	2039						1/1/2023		
57 Geng Shen	2040								
58 Xin You	2041								
59 Ren Xu	2041								
60 Gui Hai	2043		5/10/22	7/9/22	9/7/22	11/6/22	1/5/23	3/6/23	5/5/23

Appendix B

Using the above table, determine the Stem and Branch of the day to determine the "open" point from the chart below. The open point is the "ruling" point and is to be used with its corresponding coupled point.

Open Point Table 1 (7:00 AM to 7:00 PM Stems 1 -30)

	7 to 9	9 to 11	11 to 13	13 to 15	15 to 17	17 to 19
1 Jia Zi	LU 7	SJ 5	SI 3	KD 6	SJ 5	BL 62
2 Yi Chou	KD 6	SP 4	GB 41	KD 6	KD 6	SJ 5
3 Bing Yin	PC 6	SP 4	SP 4	GB 41	KD 6	LU 7
4 Ding Mao	SP 4	GB 41	KD 6	SP 4	GB 41	BL 62
5 Wu Chen	KD 6	LU 7	GB 41	SI 3	KD 6	SJ 5
6 Ji Si	SJ 5	SP 4	GB 41	KD 6	SP 4	GB 41
7 Geng Wu	KD 6	LU 7	GB 41	KD 6	KD 6	SJ 5
8 Xin Wei	GB 41	KD 6	KD 6	SJ 5	BL 62	KD 6
9 Ren Shen	GB 41	KD 6	SP 4	GB 41	KD 6	KD 6
10 Gui You	GB 41	KD 6	SP 4	SJ 5	BL 62	KD 6
11 Jia Xu	SJ 5	SP 4	BL 62	PC 6	SP 4	GB 41
12 Yi Hai	KD 6	SJ 5	BL 62	KD 6	KD 6	SP 4
13 Bing Zi	SI 3	KD 6	KD 6	SJ 5	BL 62	PC 6
14 Ding Chou	KD 6	SP 4	GB 41	KD 6	SP 4	SJ 5
15 Wu Yin	LU 7	SI 3	KD 6	KD 6	SJ 5	BL 62
16 Ji Mao	GB 41	BL 62	KD 6	SJ 5	BL 62	KD 6
17 Geng Chen	KD 6	SJ 5	SI 3	KD 6	PC 6	SP 4
18 Xin Si	BL 62	KD 6	KD 6	SP 4	GB 41	KD 6
19 Ren Wu	KD 6	LU 7	GB 41	KD 6	LU 7	SJ 5
20 Gui Wei	KD 6	SJ 5	BL 62	GB 41	KD 6	SP 4
21 Jia Shen	KD 6	KD 6	LU 7	SI 3	KD 6	SJ 5
22 Yi You	BL 62	KD 6	SJ 5	BL 62	GB 41	KD 6
23 Bing Xu	BL 62	PC 6	PC 6	SP 4	GB 41	KD 6
24 Ding Hai	KD 6	SJ 5	BL 62	KD 6	SJ 5	SP 4
25 Wu Zi	PC 6	SP 4	BL 62	GB 41	KD 6	LU 7
26 Ji Chou	SP 4	SJ 5	BL 62	KD 6	SJ 5	BL 62
27 Geng Yin	SJ 5	BL 62	KD 6	SJ 5	SP 4	GB 41
28 Xin Mao	KD 6	SP 4	SJ 5	BL 62	KD 6	SJ 5
29 Ren Chen	KD 6	SJ 5	SI 3	KD 6	SJ 5	SP 4
30 Gui Si	KD 6	SP 4	GB 41	BL 62	KD 6	SJ 5

Open Point Table 2 (7:00 AM to 7:00 PM Stems 31 -60)

	7 to 9	9 to 11	11 to 13	13 to 15	15 to 17	17 to 19
31 Jia Wu	LU 7	SJ 5	SI 3	KD 6	SJ 5	BL 62
32 Yi Wei	KD 6	SP 4	GB 41	KD 6	KD 6	SJ 5
33 Bing Shen	LU 7	SI 3	SI 3	KD 6	SJ 5	BL 62
34 Ding You	BL 62	KD 6	SJ 5	BL 62	KD 6	KD 6
35 Wu Xu	KD 6	LU 7	GB 41	SI 3	KD 6	SJ 5
36 Ji Hai	SJ 5	SP 4	GB 41	KD 6	SP 4	GB 41
37 Geng Zi	KD 6	LU 7	GB 41	KD 6	KD 6	SJ 5
38 Xin Chou	GB 41	KD 6	KD 6	SJ 5	BL 62	KD 6
39 Ren Yin	SJ 5	BL 62	KD 6	SJ 5	BL 62	GB 41
40 Gui Mao	SJ 5	BL 62	KD 6	KD 6	SP 4	GB 41
41 Jia Chen	SJ 5	SP 4	BL 62	PC 6	SP 4	GB 41
42 Yi Si	KD 6	SJ 5	BL 62	KD 6	KD 6	SP 4
43 Bing Wu	SI 3	KD 6	KD 6	SJ 5	BL 62	PC 6
44 Ding Wei	KD 6	SP 4	GB 41	KD 6	SP 4	SJ 5
45 Wu Shen	BL 62	PC 6	SJ 5	SP 4	GB 41	KD 6
46 Ji You	KD 6	KD 6	SP 4	GB 41	KD 6	SP 4
47 Geng Xu	KD 6	SJ 5	SI 3	KD 6	PC 6	SP 4
48 Xin Hai	BL 62	KD 6	KD 6	SP 4	GB 41	KD 6
49 Ren Zi	KD 6	LU 7	GB 41	KD 6	LU 7	SJ 5
50 Gui Chou	KD 6	SJ 5	BL 62	GB 41	KD 6	SP 4
51 Jia Yin	BL 62	GB 41	PC 6	SP 4	GB 41	KD 6
52 Yi Mao	SP 4	GB 41	KD 6	SP 4	SJ 5	BL 62
53 Bing Chen	BL 62	PC 6	PC 6	SP 4	GB 41	KD 6
54 Ding Si	KD 6	SJ 5	BL 62	KD 6	SJ 5	SP 4
55 Wu Wu	PC 6	SP 4	BL 62	GB 41	KD 6	LU 7
56 Ji Wei	SP 4	SJ 5	BL 62	KD 6	SJ 5	BL 62
57 Geng Shen	GB 41	KD 6	SP 4	GB 41	SI 3	KD 6
58 Xin You	SJ 5	BL 62	GB 41	KD 6	SP 4	GB 41
59 Ren Xu	KD 6	SJ 5	SI 3	KD 6	SJ 5	SP 4
60 Gui Hai	KD 6	SP 4	GB 41	BL 62	KD 6	SJ 5

Glossary

bā guà 八卦 eight diagrams

chǐ 尺 Chinese foot, roughly equivalent to 12 inches

chòng mài 冲脉 thoroughfare vessel; one of the Eight Extraordinary
   vessels

cùn 寸 Chinese inch

dà zhōu tiān 大周天 large heavenly circuit; more encompassing the
   the small heavenly circuit

dài mài 带脉 girdling or belt vessel; one of the Eight Extraordinary
   vessels

dào 道 a way, path, process. The ultimate reality of the universe.

dào jiào 道教 Daoism

díchōng 地冲 earth's thoroughfare; alternate name for KD 1

díhù 地戶 earth's door; alternate name for Ren 1

dū mài 督脉 governing vessel; one of the Eight Extraordinary vessels

gān zhī 干支 sexagenarian cycle or cycle of 60

gōng néng 功能 function, capability

hé chē 河车 river chariot, aka "microcosmic orbit"

hé tú 河图 river diagram

hòu tiān 后天 post-heaven (as opposed to pre-heaven)

hún 魂 ethereal, immortal soul; housed in the Liver; element wood

jiājǐguān 夾脊關 spinal handle gate; second of the three gates,
   located at Du 11

jīng 精 essence

jīng luò 经络 channels and collaterals; the acupuncture channels body

jiǔ gōng tú 九宫 nine palaces

Ling Gui Ba Fa 灵龟八法 Eight Methods of the Sacred Turtle

liǎng yí 两仪 two paths, two intentions (yin/yang before separation)

lóng guī 龙龟 dragon turtle

lóng mǎ 龙马 dragon horse

luò shū 洛书 luo river scroll

mìng 命 life

nèi dān 内丹 internal alchemy

nèi jiā 内家 an internal or "soft" martial art

níwán 泥丸 muddy pellet (brain)

nìxíng 逆行 "inverting the course"

pò 魄 corporeal soul, mortal soul; housed in the Lungs; element metal

qì 氣 energy, breath, vitality

qìgōng 气功 energy cultivation

qí jīng bā mài 奇經八脈 the Eight Extraordinary Vessels

rèn mài 任脉 conception vessel; one of the Eight Extraordinary vessels

sān guān 三關 three gates or barriers which are to be opened

sān bǎo 三宝 three treasures

shén 神 spirit, conscious mind; housed in the Heart; element fire

shí èr zhī 十二枝 12 terrestrial branches; the energy cycle of earth

shí tiāngān 十天干 10 celestial stems; the energy cycle of heaven

shùnhuà 顺化 "continuing transformation," "going along"

tài jí 太极 Supreme Ultimate

tàijíquán 太極拳 Supreme Ultimate boxing; an internal martial art

tiānjīng 天睛 celestial eye; alternate name for Yintang

tiānmén 天門 heaven's gate; alternate name for Du 20

wài jiā 外家 external or "hard" martial arts

wàn wù 萬物　all living things

wàng 望 to look towards or gaze into the distance

wěilǘguān 尾閭關 caudal funnel gate; located in the sacral area

wú jì 無極 limitless, boundless

wǔ shèn 五神　five spirits

wú wéi 无为 non-doing, the natural course of action

wǔ xíng 五行　five phases

wù zhì 物质 matter, substance

xiān tiān 先天 pre-heaven

xiǎo zhōu tiān 小周天 small heavenly circuit; see "hé chē"

xìng 性 nature

xíng xì quán 太極拳 Mind-Intention boxing; an internal martial art

xuè 穴 cave, cavity, hole; acupuncture point

yáng 阳　male principle, active

yáng qiào mài 阳跷脉 yang motility vessel; one of the Eight
　　　　　　　　Extraordinary vessels

yáng wéi mài 阳维 脉 yang linking vessel; one of the Eight
　　　　　　　　Extraordinary vessels

yì 意 intention, thought; housed in the Spleen; element earth

yīn 阴　female principle, passive

yīn qiào mài 阴跷脉 yin motility vessel; one of the Eight
　　　　　　　　Extraordinary vessels

yīn wéi mài 阴维 脉 yin linking vessel; one of the Eight
　　　　　　　　Extraordinary vessels

yǒu wéi 有为 doing (as opposed to non-doing)

yúzhěnguān 玉枕關 jade pillow gate; third of the three gates , located at Du 17

yǔ zhòu xué 宇宙学　cosmology

yuán 元　original, primary

zàng fǔ 脏腑 12 internal organs; 6 yin, 6 yang

zhì 志　　aspiration, ambition, will; housed in the Kidneys; element water

Reference Notes

1. Carrol, Lewis. *Alice's Adventures in Wonderland.* Chapter Five. London: Macmillan and Co, 1865.

2. Feng, Gia-Fu. *Tao Te Ching.* Chapter One. New York: Random House, 1972.

3. Sima Qian, trans. by Burton Watson. *Shǐjì* 史记, *Records of the Grand Historian.* Columbia University Press, 3rd edition, 1995.

4. Li, Dun J. *The Civilization of China, From the Formative Period to the Coming of the West.* Chapter One, Part Two. New York: Charles Scribner's & Sons, 1975.

5. Pregadio, Fabrizio. *The Seal of the Unity of the Three.* Number 10, lines 10-13. Mountain View, CA: Golden Elixir Press, 2011.

6. Orsborn, John. *Qīng Jìng Jīng* 清靜經 – *The Classic of Clarity and Stillness.* Personal Translation, 2022

7. Cleary, Thomas. *Understanding Reality, A Taoist Alchemical Classic.* Part One, number 14. Honolulu: University of Hawaii Press, 1987.

8. Wang Mu. *Foundations of Internal Alchemy: The Taoist Practice of Neidan.* Page 110. Mountain View, CA: Golden Elixir Press, 2011.

9. Orsborn, John. *Qīng Jìng Jīng* 清靜經 – *The Classic of Clarity and Stillness.* Personal Translation, 2022

10. Gu He Dao. *History of Chinese Medicine (Zhong Guo Yi Xue Shi Lue).* Taiyuan: Shanxi's Peoples Publishing House, 1979

11. Deadman, Peter and Mazin Al-Khafaji. *A Manual of Acupuncture.* Page 17. Vista, CA: Eastland Press, 2001

12.   Chace, Charles and Miki Shima. *An Exposition on the Eight Extraordinary Vessels: Acupuncture, Alchemy, & Herbal Medicine.* Part One, Chapter C, page 20. Seattle: Eastland Press, 2010.
13.   Zhang, Zhongjing. *Treatise on Febrile Disease Caused by Cold with 500 Cases.* Clause 9, note 1. Beijing: New World Press, 1993.
14.   Yang, Jizhou, trans. by Lorraine Wilcox. *The Great Compendium of Acupuncture and Moxibustion (Zhen Jiu Da Cheng Volume 5).* Portland: The Chinese Medicine Database, 2010.
15.   Liu, Lihong. *Classical Chinese Medicine.* Chapter One, page 29. Hong Kong: The Chinese University Press, 2019.
16.   Orsborn, John. *Qīng Jìng Jīng* 清靜經 – *The Classic of Clarity and Stillness.* Personal Translation, 2022
17.   Cleary, Thomas. *The Book of Balance and Harmony.* Chapter Five. New York: North Point Press, 1989.
18.   Chace, Charles and Miki Shima. *An Exposition on the Eight Extraordinary Vessels: Acupuncture, Alchemy, & Herbal Medicine.* Chapter 6 (quoted by Li Shi-Zhen from Zhang Boduan's *Eight Vessel Scripture*, now lost). Seattle: Eastland Press, 2010.
19.   Wu, Jing-Nuan. *Ling Shu or The Spiritual Pivot.* Honolulu: University of Hawaii Press, 1993.

John Orsborn, A.P., D.O.M. is a National Board Certified Acupuncture Physician and Doctor of Oriental medicine, licensed in the state of Florida. He owns Tao of Wellbeing Acupuncture Clinic LLC in Bradenton, Fl where he has practiced for over 15 years. He is also a former Adjunct Professor at East West College of Natural Medicine in Sarasota, Fl., where he taught for 21 semesters. Dr. John has given seminars on Daoist acupuncture techniques and Medical Qigong, and for 10 years he taught Taiji and Qigong to cancer patients at the Center for Building Hope in Sarasota. His undergraduate studies were in Chinese philosophy, which he has studied for over 40 years. Dr. John utilizes his knowledge of Daoist philosophy to enhance and further understand the classical texts of Chinese medicine and his increase his understanding of classical acupuncture.